Boost Your Energy Levels

60 Natural Ways to Get Rid of Fatigue, Dizziness, Weakness, And Lack of Motivation

BY

KIM HILTON

Table of Contents

Introduction

Everybody wants and needs to accomplish a particular goal in a little span of time, but less and less people are able to achieve their goals due to the stress and distraction of the fast-world. The go-getters have developed different strategies of increasing and boosting energy to begin something and to last longer on a task without the need for constant rest. When you have a great energy level you won't need a lot of motivation in order to start up a task. You can just decide to pursue a goal and never stop until you reach a significant achievement.

The energy you need to accomplish things faster include both the physical, the mental and the emotional. You need to work on these three areas in order to reach a definite goal and to perform effectively. Natural ways of boosting energy exclude the use of drugs or caffeine.

In fact, caffeine or drugs are not the best ways to boost energy since they have greater side effects. In order to stay productive and healthy for a long period of time, powerful ways to boost your energy level has been well elaborated in this book.

"Take care of the body and give it the nourishment it deserves. This body is the only body you have."

CHAPTER 1: Key-starter Activities

Have sex

Studies have shown that sex does not only improve our mental and emotional energy levels but it also helps to stay focus and concentrated for a longer period of time. All the cobwebs of emotions and distraction of the opposite sex will be eliminated and you will become highly productive.

Get some sleep

Get enough sleep before you begin any creative journey. Forget about the notion that to be successful you only need 5 hours sleep. Yes, you might only need to sleep for 5 hours in the night but make sure you compensate these hours in the day time.

Really dress

When you dress to kill, you will have the definite motivation to kill. Your dressing as a whole affects your motivation to do or not to do. You are giving yourself a natural energy boost because you will look the part, and therefore no further motivation is needed.

Always finish things

Develop of a habit of finishing things before you begin the next. Finishers are always finisher because they have long ago developed such habit of finishing things. Getting things done is not a gift but a habit to be developed and maintained. It is a mental arrangement.

Go for the unfamiliar

Always be eager to try something new. People with constant motivation tend to have wider experience of activities. Do not be afraid of trying something new. It won't only improve you experience, it will improve your mental and physical muscles.

Sit up

Your working desk is not for nap or any other extracurricular activity. Since we are going natural, you are not even allowed to take some coffee on your desk. So let the primary activity that will be carried out on your desk be the task at hand.

Challenge first

Contrary to the normal rules of getting things done, start with a difficult task and descend to the simpler ones. You need all the energy you need for the most challenging tasks.

Go for interests

When having a conversation, talk to people with the same mind-set and motivation. Talk to people about your work, task or goals. Talk about your passion with other people, and the conversation will bring about the fashion in its practical form.

CHAPTER 2: Avoid Energy Drainers

Some people will drain your energy without actually making you do anything. These type of people include complainers and doubters. Stay away from them in order to maintain your energy level.

Lean on purpose

Always have something to achieve in accomplishing a task. Let your purpose be a driving force and a reason to wake up every morning chasing that goal that matter.

Go herbal

Herbal supplements provide natural energy boost and they are surprisingly more effective and healthier than the chemicals or drugs we take to boost our energy levels. Things like Maitake, Gutu kola, bee pollen, and ginseng will replace all chemical boosters.

Lose weight

Perform exercises and eat simple foods that will help you to loss some pounds. Do not go hard on yourself just drink a lot of water, exercise more and avoid fatty foods.

Work on your attitude

Firstly, stop being negative about the task you are about to accomplish. You may not like the task or be completely equipped for the job, but never underestimate the power of a simple positive thought.

Wear bright colors

Studies on mood stimulation have proved that white or bright cloths project positive mood to people, and then that positive feeling is being projected back. It is like smiling at people and people smiling back at you. You get the drill?

Change your socks

You probably heard this before because it's an old trick that still works. The aim is to feel fresh and be ready to continue on the same energy level. Change your socks midway through your working hours.

Have a clear nose

Clear stuffy nose in order to feel light and alert. Stuffy nose can make you feel cranky or tired. Use saline solution to cleanse your nasal passages blocked by sinuses caused by allergies.

Stay hydrated

A simple rule that most people forget. Anytime you feel weak and fatigued, just take a sip of some clean water. You don't need to drink a lot to keep you distracted as you pee every 10 minutes. Just stay hydrated to stay awake.

Aromatherapy and incense

Use aromatherapy essential oils in your bath in order to stimulate your brain positively. You can use vaporizer, or massage oil as well. Essential oils include, black pepper, basil, rosemary, pine, peppermint, lemongrass, lime, lemon, ginger, fir, eucalyptus, cypress, clove, cinnamon, and

bergamot.

CHAPTER 3: Things You Take into Your Body

Go for vitamins

The proper vitamins include vitamin B12, thiamine, folic acid, and pantothenic acid, all in the family of B vitamins. Other important vitamins include niacin, riboflavin, selenium, vitamin C, and vitamin D.

Cut down on energy drinks and coffee

Coffee can give you the instant energy to perform task instantly but long term use may bring about fatigue. And you may not be able to work without the usage. If you can't cut down completely, drink only one cup a day.

Choose lean protein

Blood sugar spikes, the reason for most dizziness, can be prevented with the intake of lean protein. Also, you will feel fuller for a longer period of time. Examples of lean protein foods include chicken breasts, lean pork, fish and other seafood.

Choose whole grains

Energy foods and whole grains contain complex carbohydrates that provide for longer energy maintenance. This is because complex carbohydrates are not easy to break down.

Eat smaller meals

Eat more frequent but smaller meals. This is to avoid the groggy feeling associated with the need for your system to digest large meals at a little amount of time.

Cut down on sugar

Sugar consumption is the major cause of energy fluctuations in the human body. If you have to take sugar, make sure you perform daily exercises to stay refreshed.

CHAPTER 4: Daily Practices

Use naps

Take few minutes' naps in-between work process to get a creative energy boost. Naps are very important to keep you refreshed and alert. In fact, with good naps you will be able to achieve double of what you suppose to achieve in a day.

Stretch

Take time to stretch after staying on the desk for an hour or so. Stretching also means taking a walk from one room to the other just to get your joints lubricated before you can continue working. Also, exercises such as yoga have provided suitable stretching mechanism you can include in your leisure time in order to get rid of fatigue.

Eliminate the habit of late night unproductive tasks

Aimless late night browsing or watching television will rob you of your sleep-time. Instead of those activities, focus on getting more sleep.

Altruism

Allow your motivation be driven from good deeds. Have the faith that by doing good and diligently, you will obtain positivity and the

right energy that will boost your happiness.

You will get satisfaction in your endeavor

and you will get to chase better things.

CHAPTER 5: Energy Conservation

Spend your energy the best way possible. Realize when you have to do something that does not require absolute productivity. Focus on the things that will turn into betterments instead of the mere need to do something. Always project your energy towards activities that provide visible benefit.

The 3 meals rule

Eat at least 3 times a day and eat at the right time. Do not skip your meal for work. Pause everything and eat first. Take care of the body and give it the nourishment it deserves. This body is the only body you have.

Exercise in the morning

Start your day with a good exercise for 30 minutes. This will require waking earlier than normal in order to energize before starting a normal day. It is important to reach an effective energy level and to get rid of all the drowsiness. Start active and you will have the most productive day.

Work on your breath

Handle stress by taking deep breathes during your work process. Sometime you may need to stop whatever you are doing just to take 30 seconds timeout to breath. This is one of the most important methods of energy conservation.

CHAPTER 6: Work On Your Organizational Skills

Keep everything in place, starting from the kind of task you are going to pursue and the elements involved in finishing those tasks. Make sure you have all the required hardware in place before you start on a task. Use minimum energy to reach your goals. Never slack for any reason.

Work on your time management skills

Your time management skill is very important also in conserving and boosting your energy level. Know when to start something and when to stop. Always work with deadlines and work daily to overcome procrastination.

The cold water trick

After having a long day or long hours of work and still need to feel energetic in order to accomplish something, splash a cold water on your face. Also wash your hands with ice cold water in order to feel alive again.

Make a plan

Plan your day according to what you want to get done. That is a perfect idea but also record everything as it is being done. Work with to-do lists all the time in order to improve organization, keep your mind busy and know where and how to spend your energy. This is a plan for wise energy management.

Take breaks

Taking breaks every 2 hours just to exercise will provide an excellent energy boost. This exercise may also involve taking a walk or jumping. The aim is to get your blood rushing, making sure that your body remain as active as your brain.

Peppermint gum

Chew sugar-free gums in order to remain alert. Advisably, peppermint gums will help you feel fresh because of the flavor and absence of sugar. Without sugar, your teeth will not rot and you will achieve maximum alertness.

The tap mechanism

Use your fingertips to tap the top of your head lightly. Do this for 5 minutes. This simple exercise helps boost energy levels.

The pressure mechanism

Place your finger tips on the top of the back of your neck and apply some pressure.

Massage this area for a few minutes and feel the energy rush.

Get cool

Stay near the window or get the Air Condition up and running in order to have a cool environment. The aim is to avoid the feeling of mental fatigue usually common by warm and airtight environment.

Just laugh

Laughing improves mood and also proves a visible boost to mental energy. Your productivity will be boosted to the roof-top once you can relax and have a good laugh.

Watching a funny video clip during your timeout is a good place to start.

Seek inspiration

Sometime you don't get inspired by sitting around waiting for an inspiration. Actually read something that will inspire you to either start something or to push even harder as you try to accomplish your goals.

The toe system

"Roll up down on your toes in order to get your circulatory system active, providing the needed oxygen throughout the body."

Go for music

Stay away from cool music if you really want to get an instant energy to do something. Go for fast beat music in order to get pushed to do something without the need to keep thinking about whether you can do it or not. Your motivation will not be determined by your skills or confidence but by the instant motivation that you will derive through the music.

Choose low carb

Low carb snacks are nutritious. You can also include fruits like grapefruits, oranges, apples and raspberries. Do as much as possible to take little of dairy products, breads and meats. The aim is to remain healthy even as you improve your energy level.

Talk to someone

When you feel down and weak, pick up that phone and call a close friend. Talk to someone you care about in order to create a good mood where there is none.

The earlobe mechanism

Pull down on your earlobes in order to stay alert and awake. The aim is to stimulate the nerve jolt that will keep you alert in order to accomplish known tasks.

CHAPTER 7: The New Habit

Go outside

Being indoors for a while can affect your mood negatively. Go outside, get some fresh air and get in touch with other human beings. Have a random conversation in order to arouse your senses of relativity.

Go bright

Turn on the lights in your room in order to stay longer on that task. It was scientifically proven that darkness enhances laziness and fatigue. You will feel the need to sleep staying longer in a dark environment. Go bright!

Go dark

The part of the brain responsible for processing information during your sleep works more efficiently when the lights are out in your bedroom. So, never sleep with the lights on. Always turn off the light to provide for active and effective processing of information and to also have better night rest.

Do not skip breakfast

Apart from starting your day with a good exercise, good food will also provide better energy to start your day like a boss.

Go nuts

Peanuts and almonds are rich in fiber and magnesium, which work in providing great energy boost. Take these nuts with half cup of water and you will be alright.

Wholegrains

Wholegrains provide long lasting fuel to help you stay energetic and active. Stay away from pasta and bread and replace your meal with wholegrains for health and energy boost.

Yogurt

More nutrients are absorbed from the food you eat when you have a healthy intestine. Yogurt has the primary function of keeping the intestines healthy. All in all, when more nutrients are absorbed, the more energy to be reserved for usage.

Skip the alcohol

Apart from preventing your body from getting enough sleep, me and you know the detrimental effect of alcohol to your system.

Skip the next alcohol, and the next, and the next.

Improve your calcium intake

Calcium works in providing higher physical endurance level. The required daily calcium level intake for an average man is about 1000mg.

Get a massage

Get a massage at least two times a month in order to get rid of soreness, headaches and anxieties.

Work on yourself confidence

One way to do this is by acknowledging your best qualities and affirming them. List down the first five things you like about yourself and say it to yourself every morning in front of the mirror.

CHAPTER 8: Natural Ways to Boost Energy Levels

Energy is very important. We cannot do anything if we are lacking in energy. Energy is the most demanded thing by the human body. And we mainly get energy through our foods, lifestyle, and state of mind.

Many people are becoming energy deficient these days. This condition has even been given a name. In natural healing, it is called chronic fatigue syndrome.

This is characterized by serious tiredness even without doing anything. Chronic stress and unhealthy diet can deplete your energy stores in the body.

This post focuses on how to increase your levels of energy naturally.

Effective Ways to Boost Your Energy Levels

1. Manage stress effectively

Stress is regarded as the "silent killer". It damages a lot of things in your body and affects your health. Stress elevates the levels of stress hormones in your body.

This would weaken your organs and reduce your levels of energy. Look for ways to manage stress effectively. Create time for rest and quality sleep. These help relieve stress and reduce the levels of stress hormones.

You can also make time for meditation, exercise, and deep breathing. All these would relieve stress and energize you.

2. Exercise

Exercises energize you. Studies have shown that 20 minutes of exercise daily increase your energy levels. It increases your metabolism and boosts your overall health.

Exercise energizes you by increasing blood flow to all your cells, tissues, and organs. This will increase the levels of oxygen in your body and flood your body with energy.

Another way exercise energizes is to eliminate toxins from your body. Toxins obstruct many metabolic processes in your body including the production of energy.

When you exercise, your body breaks down a lot of toxins and expels them through sweat. This cleanses your body and promotes the production of energy.

Exercises that can help you are walking, cycling, swimming, jogging, etc. aerobic exercises that make you take in more oxygen are good in energizing you. But don't go above your limit. Listen to your body.

Always remember to drink enough water after exercising. Your body has lost water through sweat, so this lost fluid has to be replaced.

3. Sunlight

Sunlight energizes. It also brightens your mood, relieves stress, moodiness, depression, and regulates the levels of your hormones. Gentle sun rays increase the activities of your blood cells.

Spend at least 30 minutes in gentle sunlight daily. You can do this during sunlight or sunset. Avoid high sunlight. Just absorb the rays of sun during these times and your energy levels will be high.

4. Quality sleep

Sleep deprivation makes you exhausted. If you skip night sleep, you will notice that you will be tired in the morning. Sometimes, you even find it difficult to control yourself.

This can affect your physical activities and even mental performance. You will be tired even without doing anything. This simply shows that sleep helps the produce sufficient energy to last us for the day.

During a state of deep sleep at night, a lot of healing and energy production takes place. When you don't sleep at night, you deprive your body of an opportunity to heal and repair and also produce energy.

Sleep energizes. So create time for sleep and don't make it a habit to skip night sleep. As an adult, you need 8 to 9 hours of night sleep. This is one of the natural things that energize you.

5. Water

Proper hydrations energizes while dehydration makes you deficient in energy. Water is used in the production of energy and a little drop in the percentage of water in your body can lead to exhaustion, fatigue, and tiredness.

After thirst and dry lips, the next common sign of dehydration is fatigue and tiredness. This is then followed by headaches and other symptoms of dehydration.

This is why you need proper hydration to prevent dehydration from happening in the first place. Your body is made up of 70 to 80% water. And you have to maintain this for energy production and optimal health.

Listen to your body and take in sufficient amount of water daily. You need more water when you exercise or indulge in strenuous physical activities. You also need more water during hot weathers.

Make sure your water is clean and free from dangerous chemicals. You can carry a bottle of water with you always. This will help you take sips at interval to avoid dehydration.

Also, increase your intake of fresh fruits and watery vegetables. They contain the purest water in nature. Avoid sugary drinks, flavored water, alcohol, and unhealthy drinks loaded with refined sugars and chemicals.

Another good way hydrate your body is to take coconut water. This drink is not only energizing, it is also therapeutic. It is called the "natural sport drink".

Another good drink to add to your diet is lemon water. Warm lemon water is a powerful energizer and also a therapeutic drink.

6. Avoid junks

Good nutrition promotes high levels of energy while bad nutrition makes you deficient in energy. This is because nutrients are used in energy metabolism and junks are void of nutrients.

They have been stripped of their nutritional qualities in the process of making them. They are also called "empty calories". Junks include processed foods, refined sugar and sugary foods and drinks, refined carbohydrates, etc.

All these can increase your energy levels in minutes but they do not last. Before you know it, your energy levels would come crashing down. This makes you weaker than before.

So, your main foods should natural and organic foods. They should be healthy. They should be more of whole grains, fruits and veggies, legumes, roots and tubers, etc.

You can eat junks and processed foods once in a while but they should not be your main food.

7. Nuts and Seeds

This class of foods is often neglected whereas they are a rich source of energy for the body. Nuts and seeds are rich in omega-3 fatty acids. The body uses this to manufacture energy.

Nuts and seeds will increase your energy levels when you add them to your diet daily. They also help to regulate hormone levels and they promote the functions of hormones.

And hormones control energy levels and physical strength. Examples of seeds and nuts to add to your daily diet are flaxseeds, chia seeds, sesame seeds, walnuts, almonds, pumpkin seeds, sunflower seeds, cashew nuts, etc.

History has it that the ancient Mayan and Aztecs warriors ate chia seeds before going to battle. They believed it made them strong and alert. Science has proven this to be true. So enjoy more seeds and nuts daily.

You can eat them alone or mix them with your diet. There are many ways to include nuts in your diet. You can find many recipes online.

8. Positive emotions

Positive emotions such joy, gratitude, happiness, peacefulness, motivation, and others increase energy. Meanwhile negative energies and emotions drain your body of energy.

Choose to focus on the positive. Dwelling on positive things and appreciating the little things that many take for granted will energize you and help you live healthier.

Don't keep anger for a long time. You have to power to refuse anger. Hatred, jealousy, envy, and other negative energies and emotions will make you weak physically. They also create health problems.

Choose to be happy, surround yourself with happy people and be genuinely happy for people.

9. Nutrients and Supplements

There are specific nutrients and supplements that are known to increase energy levels. I will be showing you the common ones which you can easily find.

Note that, the best way to get nutrients is through your diet and not through supplements. Supplements increase your risks of toxicity if they are taken for a long time.

So, they should be taken for a short while to avoid toxicity. It is difficult to get toxicity through diet. You get these nutrients naturally by increasing your intake of foods rich in the particular nutrients.

Supplements should only be taken when prescribed by a doctor. Don't take it on your own to increase energy. If you must, meet a doctor to prescribe a good supplement for you.

Some of the nutrients that energize the body are:

- **B vitamins:** These are vitamin B1 to B12. Another name for B vitamin is "energy vitamins". The most complex of this is B12. It is one of the best vitamins taken for energy levels.

  These energy vitamins support the production of energy in your body. They keep all your blood cells healthy, active, and happy. The first sign of a deficiency in these vitamins, especially vitamin B12 is fatigue and general weakness.

  Your body cannot save extra amount of B12 because it is water-soluble. This means you have to get it from foods or from supplements.

  Natural sources of vitamin B12 are: medicinal mushrooms, nutritional milks, plant-based milk from seeds and nuts. You can also get B12 from organic animal products like eggs, seafood, meat, and dairy.

10. Vegetable smoothies

Fresh vegetable juice is an energy drink. It shocks your body in a good way and this energizes you. If you want instant energy, you can juice this smoothie to remove the fiber.

Your digestive system consumes a lot of energy trying to digest fiber. When you remove the fiber, your body would have enough energy almost instantly.

Vegetable juice or smoothies contain lots of vitamins and minerals which are needed for energy production. These nutrients supply energy to all the cells of your body.

If you feel a sickness, coming on, the best way to stop it in its tack and increase your energy is to drink vegetable smoothies. Avoid the ones sold in the shops and make yours at home.

The ones sold in the shop are loaded with sugar, preservatives, and other unhealthy chemicals. Instead of energizing you, these commercially prepared vegetable juices will deplete your energy levels and make you feel exhausted or even worse.

11. Herbs

Herbs are medicinal plants that are taken to treat various illnesses. They are many ways to take herbs. Some are taken in pill forms, some are taken in the form of teas, and some are taken in the form of teas.

Most herbs are used in cooking because they are natural spices. They improve the taste and aroma of foods. You can add herbs to your meals during preparation.

Common energizing herbs you should know are:

- Ginger
- Green tea extract
- Ashwangandha
- Mushrooms
- Suma roots
- Basil leaves
- Astragalus
- Kola nut
- Moringa
- Garlic

Herbal teas to take for increased energy levels and alertness are:

- Ginger and lemon tea
- Moringa tea
- Green tea

- Yerba mate tea

- Black tea

- Licorice root tea

- Peppermint tea

- Chamomile tea

- Turmeric tea

12. Essential oils

The use of essential oils and aromatherapy is a good way to increase your mental functions and stimulate your mind. They also increase the levels of your energy and they are powerful enough to treat weaknesses and tension headaches.

Peppermint essential oil energizes. It is one of the most common oils used in aromatherapy. Diffuse peppermint oil in your home or put a few drops on your wrist and inhale it.

You can add few drops of this oil to your shower to give you an early morning burst of energy.

Conclusion

Your lifestyle and diet affect your energy level and overall health. Choose a healthy and active lifestyle and also choose a healthy diet to junk and processed foods and you will have lots of energy to carry on your daily activities.

Exhaustion, fatigue, or tiredness happens when you are faulting in one of these or both. Nutritional deficiencies are one of the leading triggers of tiredness and lack of energy.

You increase your risk for nutritional deficiency when you replace healthy and nutritious foods with junks. Don't make junks and processed foods your main meal if you don't want to be lacking in energy.

Make healthy foods your main meals. Don't make it a lifestyle to skip night sleep. You need quality sleep for energy metabolism. Also, short naps in the afternoon also help energize you.

It is with a great honor to provide the needed information that will help you to stay healthy and fit. Pick 10 out of these listed tips and try them for two weeks. Come back, pick more and implement. The aim is to cultivate healthy habits that will help you reach an optimum energy level. These habits should become part of you as a person, even as you boost your health level to the utmost.